The Dementia Patients Guide:

A guide to effectively managing all forms of behavioral changes in dementia.

By

Faviola R. Johnson

TABLE OF CONTENTS

INTRODUCTION

Congratulations on taking up this book if you are a dementia caregiver. I'm delighted to have you here. Dementia disease impacts not only the person diagnosed with it but particularly the caregiver and the entire family. The most difficult issue linked with dementia is the daily struggle to discover that part of the person that is still there and to connect emotionally with the person that remains to fully enjoy that experience, however fleeting it may be.

The task is to give comfort, reassurance, and love regularly, patiently, and freely. Consider love as a verb rather than merely a noun. Many family caregivers, like you, are committed to providing home care for loved ones in the later stages of dementia for as long as possible.

Some families are unable to maintain a high quality of home-based care because they lack the personal care skills required for dementia care.

Others quit because they did not anticipate or plan for the care-related issues that arose. Other carers risk their health to fulfill their commitment to home-based care, making it impossible for them to continue.

It is difficult to sustain the commitment to keep someone with dementia at home throughout the illness, but with adequate planning, assistance, solid information, and the right attitude, prolonged home-based care is truly achievable.

This book takes an in-depth look into dementia caregiving. A comprehensive practical tip to help you in the day-to-day care of the person with dementia disease. We'll look at the various causes of dementia and how they can be diagnosed and treated. It also highlights the most common changes that people with dementia go through, as well as how you can best support them. This guide also provided information on the Right approach to maintaining good Diets and Nutrition with dementia. Suitable activities and exercise for people with dementia are also highlighted.

Your mental stability is the most critical factor in your loved one's quality of life. So, we'll also discuss about your health.

I present bulleted lists of actions you can take for each topic and inform you that you have options regardless of whether it feels like you don't.

I've cared for dementia patients and their families. Specializing in this care meant becoming a certified dementia educator.

If there's one thing, I've learned in my years of caring for people with dementia, it's that we are more than just our brains. Thought and language are produced by the brain, but they do not tell the entire story of who we are. We are conscious beings. We have a soul that is immune to physical sicknesses.

Remember that no matter how far away your loved one appears to be, they are still here, they care about you and also understand you're doing everything you can, and nothing is going to change that. Just that, they're unable to express themselves in the ways they once did, but dementia cannot eliminate that fact.

When you believe your loved one is no longer with you, remember their soul. Remember their principles, their life priorities, and the emotions you both shared. Dementia cannot destroy any of these things because they exist beyond space and time. Keep them safe.

I wish you the best of luck on your caregiving journey. You have my highest regard. Hold on to the person your loved one is today. And never doubt that the heart remembers what the head cannot.

CHAPTER ONE

WHAT PRECISELY IS DEMENTIA?

A brain disease called dementia causes a person's cognitive ability to decline. The intricate organ known as the brain is necessary for mental and behavioral functions. The inability to understand or remember new information is a common consequence of brain illnesses. Dementia is one instance. A person with dementia has a gradual decline in their cognitive ability over years or months. Many cognitive abilities are impacted by dementia, including memory, language, attention, orientation, judgment, and planning.

Dementia signs and symptoms

When once-healthy neurons (nerve cells) in the brain stop functioning, lose connections with other brain cells, and eventually die, dementia symptoms arise. As people age, they may lose some neurons, but those who have dementia lose a lot more. Depending on the kind, dementia has different indications and symptoms.

- Short-term memory loss is the most common symptom that the affected individual, their family, or other people notice right away. Examples include forgetting previous conversations and where one places things around the house. The ability to function properly in daily life is impaired by these problems, which occur often (several times per day over several months or years) in dementia.

- Withdrawal from interests or social events; anxiety or sadness; trouble remembering to take prescriptions; trouble following directions, such as straying and getting lost in a familiar neighborhood, are all warning signs.

- Having trouble reading and writing

- Having delusions or paranoia

- Having trouble speaking, interpreting, and expressing thoughts

- It takes longer to finish daily routine tasks

- Acting rashly and insensitive to other people's feelings

- Dizziness and trouble moving

As people age, dementia can strike those with intellectual and developmental problems, and in these cases, it might be more difficult to identify the signs. It's important to assess an individual's current abilities and monitor any changes over time that can point to dementia.

THE CAUSES OF DEMENTIA

Dementia is caused by a brain disease or an injury to the brain. It can be caused by medical disorders that begin elsewhere in the body. A person's thinking can be affected by an irregular heart rhythm, which can cause a blood clot to develop in the heart, travel to the brain, and block blood flow to a brain region. Some dementia-causing disorders begin in the brain. Alzheimer's disease is one of the most common, affecting around 5 million people in the United States. The risk of Alzheimer's disease increases with age. Dementia typically develops when the brain is afflicted by two or more prevalent aging disorders, such as Alzheimer's disease and stroke.

Additional illnesses that can result in dementia or symptoms resembling dementia include

- Normal pressure hydrocephalus, which is an abnormal build-up of CSF fluid in the brain

- Creutzfeldt-Jakob disease, a rare neurological ailment

- Huntington's illness, a degenerative, hereditary brain condition

- Delirium, an abrupt condition of confusion and disorientation

- HIV-associated dementia is a rare disease that develops when HIV spreads to the brain

- Chronic traumatic encephalopathy is brought on by repetitive traumatic brain damage.

Furthermore, serious memory deficits that mimic dementia can be brought on by medical conditions such as tumors, vitamin deficiencies, drug side effects, and thyroid, kidney, or liver issues. Several dementia symptom reasons are curable or perhaps preventable. For example, normal pressure hydrocephalus usually goes away with therapy.

The symptoms of dementia might be identical, which could make a correct diagnosis difficult. Nonetheless, a comprehensive diagnosis is necessary to get the right therapy.

Does memory loss indicate the onset of dementia?

One prevalent misconception regarding memory loss is that it invariably indicates dementia in oneself or a loved one. Several things can induce memory loss. Memory loss alone is not generally a sign of dementia.

It's also true that as people age, their memories tend to change in specific ways because certain brain neurons naturally die. On the other hand, this kind of memory loss does not impair functionality, thus daily tasks are not hindered.

Dementia reduces your ability to function. Dementia is more than merely forgetting where you placed your keys. Individuals suffering from dementia could forget why they have keys. Dementia does not usually get worse with age.

What are the various kinds of dementia?

Dementia is caused by a progressive and permanent loss of neurons and brain function driven by a variety of neurodegenerative illnesses and causes.

It is typical for some neurons in the brain to die as we age. People suffering from dementia, on the other hand, suffer significantly more loss. Many neurons cease working, lose connections to other brain cells, and finally die. Symptoms may be modest initially but gradually worsen over time.

Dementias are classified into three categories

1. Primary (diseases and disorders characterized by dementia as the primary sickness).

2. Secondary dementia (dementia caused by another disease or condition).

3. Reversible dementia-like symptoms induced by other diseases or conditions.

PRIMARY DEMENTIA

The following are examples of primary dementia:

Alzheimer's disease: The most prevalent kind of dementia is Alzheimer's disease. when the brain accumulates excessive amounts of the protein's tau and amyloid. These proteins obstruct the nerve cells in your brain from communicating with one another. As more nerve cells die, the death of a nerve cell spreads from its original location. Alzheimer's disease symptoms worsen over time.

Everyone is affected differently by Alzheimer's disease. However, several early symptoms are common such as Cognitive symptoms include mental decline, difficulty thinking and understanding, evening confusion, delusion, disorientation, forgetfulness, making things up, mental confusion, difficulty concentrating, inability to create new memories, inability to do simple maths, or inability to recognize common things.

Behavioral symptoms include aggression, agitation, problems with self-care, irritation, meaningless repetition of own words, personality changes, lack of inhibition, or roaming and getting lost are all examples of behavioral symptoms. Anger, apathy, general dissatisfaction, loneliness, or mood swings

Psychological symptoms: Depression, delusion, or paranoia.

Whole-body: Loss of appetite or restlessness, as well as walking difficulties, occur later in the disease.

An individual with Alzheimer's disease will need more assistance with everyday tasks as the illness worsens. The majority of people affected by Alzheimer's disease are older adults; up to 10% of those over 65 and roughly 50% of those over 85 are affected. One important risk factor is a person's family history. Between 60% and 80% of dementia patients have this kind of dementia.

Vascular Dementia: Vascular dementia is the second most frequent kind of dementia. It is caused by illnesses like as strokes or atherosclerosis, which block and damage blood arteries in the brain or disrupt the flow of blood and oxygen to the brain.

Symptoms include memory problems, disorientation, and difficulty focusing and completing tasks. The decrease might happen gradually (after a series of mini-strokes) or suddenly (after a big stroke). Diabetes, hypertension, and increased cholesterol levels are all risk factors. 15% to 25% of dementia individuals have vascular dementia.

Lewy Body Dementia: This dementia is characterized by the aberrant accumulation of proteins alpha-synuclein known as Lewy bodies in the nerve cells of the brain. Lewy bodies hurt nerve cells.

Symptoms include movement and balance issues, changes in sleep patterns, memory loss, planning and problem-solving difficulties, and visual hallucinations and delusions. Lewy Body dementia affects 5% to 10% of dementia patients.

Frontotemporal dementia (FTD): This type of dementia is caused by damage to the brain's frontal and temporal lobes. The damage is linked to aberrant levels or types of the protein tau and TDP-43.

It alters social behavior, and personality, and/or leads to a loss of linguistic skills (speaking, understanding, or forgetting the meaning of common words) or physical coordination. Frontotemporal dementia is a prevalent cause of early dementia, most commonly affecting adults between the ages of 45 and 64. Frontotemporal dementia accounts for 5% to 6% of all dementia.

Mixed dementia: The existence of two or more dementia types characterizes this. The most frequent pairings are vascular dementia and Alzheimer's disease. Adults over 80 years old are more likely to experience it. Since some dementia symptoms may be more obvious than others and/or many symptoms of each kind overlap, diagnosis is frequently challenging. Compared to people with only one form of dementia, people with mixed dementia decline more quickly.

SECONDARY DEMENTIA

Different types of dementia due to different diseases and circumstances include:

Huntington's disease: This brain illness is caused by a single faulty gene. The disease causes a breakdown in your brain's nerve cells, resulting in problems with body movement control, as well as difficulties with thinking, decision-making, and memory, as well as personality changes.

Parkinson's disease: A lot of people with Parkinson's disease develop dementia in their later stages.

Symptoms include difficulty thinking and remembering, hallucinations and delusions, depression, and difficulty speaking.

Creutzfeldt-Jakob disease: This is a rare infective brain disease that affects around one in a million people. The condition is caused by prions, which are aberrant proteins in your brain. These prions aggregate and destroy brain nerve cells. Confusion, behavioral changes, agitation, depression, and difficulties with thinking, remembering, communicating, planning, and/or judging are some of the symptoms.

Wernicke-Korsakoff syndrome: The cause of Wernicke-Korsakoff syndrome is a severe thiamine deficiency (vitamin B1) deficit in the brain. This can cause bleeding in memory-related parts of your brain. It is most usually caused by alcoholism; however, it can also be caused by starvation and persistent illness. Double vision, lack of motor coordination, trouble processing information, acquiring new abilities, and remembering things are all symptoms.

Traumatic brain injury (TBI): This damage can be caused by repeated impacts to the head. Football players, fighters, veterans, and people who have been in auto accidents are the groups most likely to experience it. Memory loss, behavioral or headaches, impaired speech, and mood swings are among indications of dementia that occur years later.

DEMENTIAS RESULTING FROM REVERSIBLE CAUSES

Some illnesses can generate dementia-like symptoms that can be treated, such as:

Normal Pressure Hydrocephalus (NPH): This illness occurs when cerebrospinal fluid (CSF) accumulates in the gaps (ventricles) of your brain. Excess accumulation is harmful to your brain. Brain trauma, brain infection, brain hemorrhage, or prior brain surgery can all result in NPH. Symptoms include poor balance, forgetfulness, difficulties focusing, mood swings, frequent stumbles, and inability to control one's urine. Your healthcare professional can drain extra fluid by surgically implanting a shunt (tube).

Deficiency in vitamins: Dementia-like symptoms can be caused by a lack of vitamin B1, B6, B12 cooper, and vitamin E in your diet.

Infections: HIV infection, syphilis, and Lyme disease are among infections that may cause symptoms associated with dementia. COVID-19 infection has been linked to symptoms such as "brain fog" and acute delirium.

Because COVID-19 infection causes inflammation and increases the risk of stroke, both short- and long-term cognitive impacts are being studied. In the elderly, urinary tract infections (UTIs) and lung infections can both produce symptoms resembling dementia. Other Cognitive issues can also be brought on by infections, fungi, and parasites that affect the brain and the nervous system in general.

Metabolic and endocrine conditions: The condition Addison's disease, Cushing's syndrome, hypoglycemia (low blood sugar), hypercalcemia (high calcium levels, commonly caused by hyperparathyroidism), liver cirrhosis, thyroid issues, exposure to heavy metals (such as arsenic or mercury), and thyroid issues are among the conditions that can cause dementia.

Medication side effects: Some medications, such as sleeping pills, anti-anxiety drugs, antidepressants, anti-seizure drugs, antiparkinson drugs, nonbenzodiazepine sedatives, narcotic pain relievers, statins, and others, can mimic dementia symptoms in some people If you experience any symptoms similar to dementia, ask your healthcare professional to evaluate your prescriptions.

Other causes include: Brain tumors and subdural hematomas, which are hemorrhages in the brain that occur between the brain's surface and its covering, which are two more reasons for dementia-like symptoms.

DEMENTIA LEVELS AND STAGES

What to anticipate when dementia is in its early, middle, and advanced stages.

Dementia is a general term used to describe a decline in cognitive function that affects language, memory, problem-solving abilities, and day-to-day functioning. Alzheimer's disease, vascular dementia, Lewy body dementia, and frontotemporal dementia exhibit varying rates of progression and individual variability.

Three progressive phases are distinguished among the seven stages of dementia:

1. Early-stage dementia. Another name for early-stage dementia is pre-dementia. At this point, a person can still live their life as they choose and may not show overt signs of memory loss or difficulty with daily duties. Age-related forgetfulness and mild dementia symptoms are comparable.

2. Middle/Moderate to advanced dementia. The symptoms of moderate dementia have a substantial impact on a person's personality and behavior. A person with middle-stage dementia will typically require full- or part-time caregiver assistance with daily activities. Other symptoms of moderate-stage dementia include considerable cognitive impairment and mood changes.

3. Severe or advanced dementia. Significant cognitive deterioration and physical incapacity are hallmarks of the final stage. Symptoms of late-onset dementia include an inability to move around without assistance, incontinence, and significant memory loss.

THE SEVEN STAGES OF DEMENTIA

Healthcare professionals utilize the Global Deterioration Scale, a comprehensive tool, to evaluate older individuals in all seven stages of dementia. Caretakers and medical professionals may predict the symptoms to anticipate at each of the seven stages of dementia as well as how quickly dementia advances in elderly individuals using this reliable method, commonly referred to as the GDS. When it comes to stage-related symptoms, a dementia stages chart can help caregivers stay on top of their loved one's health.

The following are the stages of cognitive decline: *Stage 1 is no cognitive impairment; Stage 2 is very mild; Stage 3 is mild; Stage 4 is moderate; Stage 5 is moderately severe; and Stage 6 is severe.*

Stage 1 Dementia: No Cognitive Impairment Is Present

Stage one dementia sometimes looks like normal mental functioning with no cognitive deterioration, despite how weird it may appear. In the initial three stages of dementia, a person usually exhibits insufficient symptoms for a diagnosis. It is important to stress, nevertheless, that the brain is still changing.

The GDS stages 1, 2, and 3 are considered to be pre-dementia stages, even though there may be some cognitive impairment present.

Stage 2 Dementia: Extremely Mild Cognitive Impairment

"Where did I put my keys?" is an example of a basic memory issue in stage 2 dementia that a loved one could have. Alternatively: "What was that person's name?" A considerable fraction of the senior population suffers from age-related forgetfulness, and carers or medical specialists may not be aware of these minors. This explains why "age-associated memory impairment" is a common term used to describe stage 2.

According to research by the British Medical Association, Professor Gary W. Small estimated that roughly 16 million Americans, or 40% of the population 65 years of age or over, suffer from age-related memory impairment. "Every year, only approximately 1% of these people succumb to dementia. Stage 2 dementia is characterized by memory loss for family members, close companions, and old acquaintances as well as disorientation from familiar objects.

Stage 3 of Dementia: Mild Cognitive Decline

Stage 3 of dementia is characterized by mild cognitive decline, also called mild cognitive impairment.

Memory and cognitive impairments that are more frequent and noticeable to family members and caregivers are signs of mild cognitive decline, sometimes referred to as mild cognitive impairment (MCI). Most of the time, stage 3 dementia does not affect day-to-day functioning.

How quickly does an elderly person's dementia advance through this stage? As per the National Institute on Ageing, within a year, 10 to 20 percent of persons 65 and older who have MCI will develop identifiable or diagnosable dementia. It is crucial to identify the signs of this stage and seek medical assistance because MCI typically precedes more severe dementia phases.

The following list of symptoms is indicative of stage 3 dementia:

- Missing events or appointments
- Losing things and mild memory loss
- Getting lost while traveling

- Decreased productivity at work

- Trouble finding the right words

- Verbal repetition

- Organization and concentration issues

- Problems with complex tasks and problem-solving.

Dementia Stage 4: Moderate Cognitive Deterioration

When a person is in stage 4 dementia, they have distinct, visible indicators of cognitive impairment as well as personality changes, both of which are significant dementia symptoms. Dementia is often not diagnosed until a person is in stage 4 or later. While the medical term for stage 4 dementia is moderate cognitive deterioration, the GDS officially classifies it as mild dementia.

Doctors and caregivers will likely see hallmark indicators of dementia progressing at this stage, such as language issues and diminished problem-solving skills, Social disengagement, Emotional mood swings, Lack of attentiveness, reduced intellectual acuity, Difficulties with everyday duties, and Forgetting recent events.

Stage 5 Dementia: Moderately Severe Cognitive Impairment

Out of the seven stages of dementia, this stage marks the start of what many experts refer to as the "mid-stage". This is the stage at which an individual may require the assistance of caregivers to do instrumental activities of daily living (IADLs) and standard ADLs like dressing or bathing. Middle-stage dementia normally lasts two to four years, with each patient progressing at their own pace.

Your loved one will most likely require more intensive help and supervision in stage 5 dementia. They remember important details about themselves, including their name and the names of their children, but they may not remember the names of their grandkids, their long-term addresses, or where they went to high school.

Symptoms of dementia in the fifth stage:

• Announced memory loss involving current events and personal information

• Nodding off/wandering

• Being disoriented and experiencing sundown syndrome;

Stage 6 Dementia: Severe Cognitive Impairment

When a person is in stage 6 dementia, they require support from a caregiver with basic daily activities including eating, going to the bathroom, and other self-care activities. At this point in their moderately severe dementia, seniors may find it difficult to interact socially, sleep properly, or act responsibly in public.

As symptoms of dementia become more complex at stage 6, you may wonder if full-time care is necessary. You can prepare by keeping track of symptoms, monitoring your loved one's capacity to perform typical activities of daily living and instrumental activities of daily living IADLs, and researching care choices such as memory care or home care.

Stage 6 dementia symptoms include:
- Disturbances in sleep
- Incontinence of the bowels or urine
- Anxiety and aggression
- Personality changes, such as delusions or psychosis

- Not being able to perform ADLs

- Significant memory loss

- Not being able to identify loved ones and caregivers

Stage 7 Dementia: Severe Cognitive Impairment

Individuals with stage 7, often known as end-stage or late-stage dementia, are incapable of taking care of themselves. In general, persons with severe dementia lose all verbal capacity and have substantially limited movement. Even if a person has end-stage dementia symptoms that indicate they are reaching the end of their life, they can live with those symptoms for months or even years.

Late-onset dementia symptoms include:

- Impairing physiological processes such as chewing, swallowing, and breathing

- Constant sleepiness

- More frequent falls and infections

- Having difficulty cognizing family and friends

- Time-shifting, or believing they are in another time

- Having difficulties eating, drinking, and swallowing

- Becoming frailer and less mobile

WHO IS AT RISK OF DEVELOPING DEMENTIA?

Aging is one factor that can increase your risk of having dementia. It is the most significant risk factor for dementia. Smoking, uncontrolled diabetes, high blood pressure, excessive alcohol consumption, and having close family members with dementia. All these factors can raise your risk of developing dementia.

CHAPTER TWO

DEMENTIA DIAGNOSIS AND MANAGEMENT

How is dementia diagnosed?

It can be difficult to confirm a dementia diagnosis. Dementia can be caused or exacerbated by a variety of diseases and circumstances. Furthermore, many of its symptoms are shared by a variety of other disorders.

- Inquire about the progression of your symptoms with your healthcare physician
- Ask about your medical history
- Review your current meds
- Inquire about your family history of illnesses, including dementia.

Your healthcare physician may also request testing such as *Laboratory Tests, Imaging Examinations, And Neurocognitive (Thinking) Tests.* Neurologists and geriatricians can diagnose dementia.

Laboratory Tests: Laboratory testing rule out a variety of disorders and conditions that could contribute to dementia, including infection, inflammation, an underactive thyroid, and vitamin deficiency (especially B12). If warranted, healthcare providers may request cerebrospinal fluid tests for the assessment of autoimmune disorders and neurodegenerative diseases.

Imaging Examinations: Your doctor may prescribe the following brain imaging tests for you:

- CT and MRI (Computerised Tomography and Magnetic Resonance Imaging). CT scans your brain with X-rays and a computer to create detailed images. MRI uses magnets, radio waves, and a computer to produce detailed images of your brain. These scans look for evidence of a stroke, hemorrhage, tumors, or fluid in the brain.

- FDG-PET Scan: This brain scan assesses brain function and cognitive impairment by analyzing how glucose is absorbed by brain tissue. It may be necessary in some situations.

Neurocognitive Testing: In neurocognitive examination, your healthcare professional evaluates your mental ability using written and computerized tests, such as:

- Problem-solving
- Learning
- Decision
- Recall
- Making a plan
- Deliberation
- The language

Psychiatric Evaluation: A psychiatric evaluation may be performed to look for evidence of depression, mood disorders, or other mental health issues that may be causing memory loss.

DEMENTIA MANAGEMENT AND TREATMENT

Dementia treatment differs depending on the individual. Before recommending a patient- and family-centered treatment plan, a doctor evaluates the medical history and individual situation. Medications may aid in thinking abilities, and mood or behavior changes, although the benefits are modest. Two groups of medications can help with memory issues, but they do not stop the disease from progressing.

It is critical to treat risk factors for stroke, such as high blood pressure and diabetes. Procedures to prevent falls or being lost are examples of safety measures. Advance directives should be written for medical and financial issues, as people with dementia frequently lose their ability to make decisions.

Other tips for excellent brain health include staying cognitively, physically, and socially active, eating nutritionally balanced meals, drinking alcohol in moderation, and getting enough high-quality sleep. Clinicians can educate family members and caregivers about dementia and assist with long-term care planning.

Is Dementia Curable?

To begin, it is necessary to understand the terms "treatable," "reversible," and "curable." All or virtually all types of dementia are treatable, which means that medication and other treatments can help you manage your symptoms. However, most types of dementia cannot be cured or reversed, and treatments are only partially helpful.

The good news is that some kinds of dementia, such as those caused by treatable conditions, can be effectively reversed. These dementia-like symptoms are the result of:

- Side effects of medications, illicit drugs, or alcohol.
- Cancerous tumors that can be removed.
- Subdural hematoma (blood accumulation beneath the outer coating of your brain caused by a head injury).
- Normal pressure hydrocephalus (cerebrospinal fluid accumulating in the brain)
- Metabolic issues, including a deficiency of vitamin B12
- Hypothyroidism, a condition caused by low thyroid hormone levels
- Hypoglycemia (a low blood sugar level)
- Depression

Dementias that are not reversible may nonetheless respond partially to drugs that treat memory loss or behavioral issues. These dementias include:

- Alzheimer's disease
- Multi-infarct dementia (vascular)
- Dementias related to Parkinson's disease and other conditions
- AIDS dementia syndrome
- Creutzfeldt-Jakob disease (CJD).

Dementia Treatments That Do Not Involve Medication

Medicines for dementia symptoms are important, but they constitute only one aspect of dementia care. Other therapies, hobbies, and caregiver assistance are essential in aiding dementia patients to live effectively.

1. Cognitive stimulation treatment (CST) involves group activities and exercises to enhance memory, problem-solving skills, and language aptitude. CST appears to benefit those with mild to moderate dementia, according to a study.

2. Cognitive rehabilitation entails working with an occupational therapist and a family member or friend to achieve a personal goal, such as learning to use a cell phone or do everyday tasks. Cognitive rehabilitation works by

encouraging you to use the parts of your brain that are functioning to help the areas that are not. It can help you cope with dementia more effectively in the early stages.

3. Reminiscence and life story work: This involves recalling memories and events from the past. Photos, treasured artifacts, and music are frequent props. A life story work is a compilation of photos, notes, and keepsakes from childhood to the present. It could be either a physical or digital book.

These approaches can sometimes be combined. There is evidence that they can increase mood and well-being. They also assist you and the people around you in focusing on your abilities and accomplishments rather than your dementia.

Drug Therapy for Dementia-Related Behaviour

A doctor may prescribe medicine if the person's behavior is detrimental to themselves or others and all other ways of soothing them have been exhausted. Speak to their GP if you want further information about pharmaceuticals to assist in managing the behavioral signs of dementia or if you are concerned about the adverse effects of medication.

What are the risks of dementia complications?

Your brain is in charge of all bodily activities. When your brain functions deteriorate, your overall health suffers. Dementia can lead to a variety of illnesses and ailments.

- Dehydration and malnutrition
- Bedsores (pressure ulcers)
- Falls and bone fractures
- Strokes
- Heart attacks
- Kidney failure
- Pneumonia and aspiration pneumonia (food particles inhaled into lungs causing pneumonia).

CHAPTER THREE

COPING WITH DEMENTIA BEHAVIOUR CHANGES: A CARERS GUIDE

Dementia can have a significant impact on the individual suffering from it. They are afraid of losing their memory and reasoning skills, but they are also afraid of losing their identity. They may also discover that they don't comprehend what's going on or why they feel out of control of what's going on around them. All of this can have an impact on their behavior.

Common Behavioural Changes

Most varieties of dementia might cause a person to change their behavior in the middle to late stages. This can be distressing for both the person with dementia and their caregivers.

Among the most prevalent behavioral changes are: Repeating the same question or conduct repeatedly, Pacing up and down, wandering, and fidgeting, wandering and fidgeting, Night-time waking and sleep disturbance, following a partner or caregiver around everywhere, Loss of self-confidence, which may show as apathy or disinterest in their usual activities etc.

1. Repeating the same question or conduct repeatedly

Repetition of the same question or conduct may indicate memory loss, in which the individual is unable to recall what they have said or done.

It can be aggravating for the caregiver, but bear in mind that the individual in question is not being deliberately difficult.

In this scenario, caregivers should:

- Be courteous and patient with them; Assist them in discovering the answer themselves. For example, if they frequently ask for the time, purchase an easy-to-read clock and keep it visible.
- Consider any underlying themes, such as the person feeling lost, and comfort them.
- Assure them that all plans are in place and they should not worry about the appointment.

2. Pacing up and down, wandering, and fidgeting

People suffering from dementia frequently exhibit restless habits such as pacing up and down, wandering out of the house, and anxious fidgeting. This stage normally does not last long.

Make sure the person has enough to eat and drink, have a daily routine including daily walks; Accompany them on a walk to the store, or consider tracking devices and alarm systems (telecare) to keep them safe; and Give them something to occupy their hands if they fidget a lot, such as worry beads or a box of items that mean something to them.

3. Night-time waking and sleep disturbance

Dementia can interrupt a person's body clock, often known as their sleep-wake cycle. Someone who is who has dementia may wake up multiple times throughout the night, unaware that it is night.

This might be especially tough for caregivers because their sleep is also affected. When this occurs, the caregiver should encourage frequent movement and exposure to sunshine; ensure that the bedroom is pleasant, provide a nightlight or blackout shades if necessary; and restrict caffeine and alcohol consumption in the evening.

4. Constantly following partner or carer around

People with dementia have feelings of insecurity and anxiety. They may "shadow" their partner or carer because they require frequent assurance that they are not alone and are safe.

They may even want people who died many years ago or request to return home without realizing they are in their own house.

This is what the caregiver should do: Have the individual with you if you are doing tasks like ironing or cooking. If they ask to go home, assure them that they are safe and protected. Instead of telling them that a particular individual passed away years ago, talk to them about that time in their lives.

5. Loss of self-esteem portrayed as indifference or disinterest in their normal activities

Dementia might make people feel insecure about going out or participating in other activities. This may appear to be a loss of interest in people or activities that they usually enjoy. Carers should keep in mind that the patient may still be interested in an activity but are concerned about how they will cope with it; reassure them that the activity, or getting there, will be simple; clearly explain where they are going and who they may be seeing; and consider simpler activities or social occasions, as, for example, participating in a conversation among a huge group of individuals may seem too challenging.

If you are caring for an individual who shows these behaviors, you must try to figure out why they are acting in this manner, which is not always easy.

It may be helpful to understand that these actions are ways for people to express their emotions. It may be good to consider other techniques for communicating with someone who has dementia.

These behaviors might not usually indicate dementia. They can be induced by dissatisfaction with not being understood or with their surroundings, something they no longer recognize as familiar but rather confusing.

HOW TO DETERMINE THE CAUSE OF THESE COMMON BEHAVIOURAL CHANGES IN DEMENTIAS

Although behavioral changes can be tough to deal with, determining if there are any triggers might be beneficial.

As an example:

- Do particular behaviors occur at specific times of day?
- Is the person's residence excessively noisy or overcrowded?
- Changes occur when individuals are asked to execute tasks they may or may not desire to do.

Keeping a diary for one to two weeks can help identify these triggers.

If the behavior change comes abruptly, the cause could be a medical problem. Constipation or disease may cause pain or discomfort for the individual.

Request an assessment to rule out or treat any underlying causes.

Establishing a lively social circle, getting regular exercise, and maintaining or discovering new hobbies that the individual loves can all help to reduce out-of-character conduct.

Managing Aggressive Behaviours in Dementias

Some patients with dementia will develop Behavioural and Psychological Symptoms of Dementia (BPSD) in the latter stages of the disease.

The following are some of the symptoms of BPSD:

- Heightened agitation
- Aggression (yelling or screaming, verbal and, in certain cases, physical abuse)
- Delusions (abnormal beliefs that are not founded on reality)
- Hallucinations (hearing or seeing nonexistent objects)

These behaviors are extremely distressing for both the carer and the person with dementia.

It is critical to request that your doctor rule out or treat any underlying reasons, such as:

- Unmanaged pain
- Untreated depression
- Infection, such as a urinary tract infection (UTI)
- medication side effects

If the individual you care for becomes hostile, try to remain cool.

Responding to the aggressive Behaviour

- Take note of what caused their distressing behavior; if you can identify these triggers, you may be able to prevent it.

- Avoid arguing or acting aggressively while they are disturbed, since this may worsen their suffering.

- Exit the room or retreat from the situation.

- Remain cool and realize that the aggressiveness, whether personal or purposeful, is caused by distress.

- Behave normally with them once they are quiet again to help you both move on.

Remember that it is not easy to be the person who supports or cares for someone who is experiencing behavioral changes. If you're having trouble, seek help from a doctor.

Carers' Needs and Support (Your Well-Being Is Important as Well)

Dementia patients might encounter mood fluctuations while managing their disease.

As dementia advances, you may feel sad, angry, fearful, or frustrated. As a caregiver, witnessing their behavior alter may be stressful and upsetting.

When caring for someone with dementia, your needs as a caregiver are just as important as the person being cared for.

- Join a local caregivers' support group or a dementia-specific association to assist you in caring for yourself.

- Join online forums and share your experiences with other caregivers.

- Take some time for yourself, but if it's tough to leave the person alone, ask if a friend, family, or member of a support group may accompany them for a bit.

- If you're feeling sad or depressed, see a doctor; you could benefit from counseling or other talking treatments.

CHAPTER FOUR

DEMENTIA DIET AND NUTRITION - CAREGIVERS APPROACH TO MAINTAINING GOOD HEALTH AND NUTRITION.

A healthy diet is essential for people with dementia's health, independence, and well-being. However, many persons with dementia may find it challenging to maintain a healthy weight. As dementia develops, eating and drinking issues become more apparent, and unwanted weight loss becomes a common problem.

Dementia is a progressive condition. It can have long-term effects on the way one eats and drinks. If you care for someone with dementia, you can assist them in maintaining a nutritious diet.

The Significance of Proper Nutrition

The individual you care for must maintain a healthy, balanced diet and engage in regular exercise.

They may become susceptible to a variety of ailments if they do not eat enough or consume toxic items.

When persons with dementia become unwell, they may become increasingly confused.

Following a dementia diagnosis, the primary goal will be to maintain a healthy weight for the individual's stature and to continue eating a good, balanced diet.

Their hunger will vary and decrease as the disease worsens. Watch out for indicators of malnutrition. This might suggest going from a standard diet to a high-calorie, high-protein one.

The purpose of nutritional treatment in the later stages of dementia is to provide the individual with the highest quality of life possible. At this stage of the illness, aggressive dietary support is usually ineffective.

Observing Changes in Eating and Drinking Habits

Observing Eating and Drinking Habits

If you care for a person with dementia, you may notice that their eating and drinking habits alter over time. This could be because of:

• Dementia progression   • Having difficulties swallowing, anxiety, sadness, loss of appetite, and lack of physical activity.

If a person's eating and drinking habits abruptly change, it could be due to:

• Dental or an oral infection   •A urinary/kidney infection; or a chest infection.   • Medicines, pain, exhaustion, and constipation.

However, not all people with dementia will have these health difficulties. If you are a carer who is concerned about the individual's health, please reach out to their primary healthcare provider.

The doctor may need to send them to a different healthcare provider.

How To Adjust to Changing Eating Habits

If you happen to detect any changes in this individual's eating and drinking habits, you may assist them by performing the following.

assisting in the creation of a tranquil environment for eating and drinking

The following can be done before a person with dementia eats or drinks:

- Ensure a quiet and distraction-free environment

- Check for dentures, glasses, and hearing aids if needed

- Clear the table of unnecessary items

- Sit as upright as possible to improve alertness

- Make use of color contrast to enable these individuals to see their food (e.g., avoid placing fish, cauliflower, and potatoes on a white plate)

- Use simple, unpatterned dishes and tablecloths

- Offer only one meal at a given moment.

How to Help Changes in Concentration Sitting at The Table to Eat A Meal

Over time, an individual experiencing dementia may struggle to concentrate and sit at a table to eat. If you care for someone with dementia, you may feel they have finished eating or They're not hungry.

They can become susceptible to a variety of diseases if they do not eat enough or consume toxic foods. When patients with dementia become unwell, their confusion may worsen.

To get them to eat and drink, you can:

They can be encouraged to eat and drink by doing the following:

- Inviting them to the table when the meal concludes so they won't have to wait; focusing their attention on the food
- Offering them the first mouthful to motivate them to feed themselves
- Reminding them to swallow every mouthful as needed
- Using gentle signs like returning the cup or cutlery to their hands
- if they forget they've already eaten or wonder when their next meal will be, reassure them and give them a snack if needed
- Sit down to dine with them; this encourages socializing and may help them keep their independence as they could imitate, you're eating habits. Just keep being supportive.

How to Assist with Changes in Coordination

It is common for a person with dementia to have difficulty feeding himself.

As eating and drinking are important for their development of independence, you must assist them at these times. Moreover, it can facilitate swallowing.

Some strategies that can be helpful include:

- Chopping food before serving it, giving them only the cutlery or cup they require
- Putting the cutlery or cup directly into their hand
- Using colorful plates and tablecloths and ensuring that the table is uncluttered
- Serving one course at a time
- Using finger foods like cheese, sandwiches, and slices of fruit or vegetables
- Giving them gentle verbal encouragement, like "smells fantastic," and placing your hand over theirs to support their meal or drink in their mouth.
- Only as a last option, think of giving them some or all of the dinner.

After losing the ability to use a spoon or fork, many people are still able to grasp a cup, and this should be promoted.

Encouraging someone to eat and drink

When the person you are taking care of begins to eat, you may help them by

- Feeding them when they are conscious and able to swallow safely; and
- When sitting down to help them eat and drink, try to be as relaxed and accommodating as possible.
- Try not to rush them
- Teaching them about what they consume
- Putting food where they can see it
- Supporting their attempts to feed themselves
- Offering cues to chew and swallow
- Sitting in front of them or slightly to their side so that you can maintain eye contact;

Helping to promote appetite

Food presentation and aroma have the power to entice people to consume. To do this, you can:

- Prepare food with a range of flavors, colors, and fragrances

- Divide different types of pureed food on the same plate, such as meat, potatoes, and vegetables; and get them to help prepare the meal or, if feasible, lay the table.

- Giving them little meals or snacks regularly and encouraging them to eat when they feel well.

- Presenting each meal individually to maintain food's warmth and appeal

- If they don't complete their supper, provide dessert.

If they wake up in the middle of the night regularly, they may be hungry.

Problems with swallowing, as well as eating and drinking

Some foods and fluids may be problematic for a person with dementia. As a result, they may spit out lumps or hold food in their mouth.

Understanding And Assisting with Swallowing Problems

Swallowing problems may become more common as dementia advances.

- Food or drink getting into the lungs rather than the stomach, sometimes causing pneumonia or chest infections
- Loss of weight
- Dehydration

The individual you are taking care of can eventually find it difficult to express whether they are hungry or thirsty. It will be necessary to monitor food and drink intake regularly to make sure they are getting adequate nutrition.

How to Adjust to Changes in Swallowing

- Providing a soft, moist diet; stay away from fibrous, hard, or dry foods like steak, bacon, and wheat bread that need a lot of chewing.
- Adding sauces or gravies to meals
- Permitting little sips of liquid

What to do when someone spits out lumps

A person with dementia may begin to spit up food.

- Steer clear of meals that have lumps, chunks, or inconsistent textures, such as soup with pieces, cookies that crumble, or anything that has skins or pips.

- Making sure the meal is consistently soft or silky

What can you do if someone forgets to swallow?

Someone with dementia can forget to swallow.

- Varying the flavors and temperatures of meals and beverages during a meal, such as savory and sweet dishes or hot and very cold foods or drinks

- Serving sips of an ice-cold beverage before a meal or in between bites

- Offering oral signals to swallow Trying to encourage swallowing by holding an empty spoon in the mouth in between bites

What Should You Do If Food Remains in Their Mouth?

A person suffering from dementia may start to keep food in their mouth after eating.

- Examining their mouth after every meal and encouraging or providing frequent denture cleaning or teeth brushing, since food particles left in the mouth can lead to bad breath and oral infections.

- Holding the person upright for a little while

- After making these attempts to aid in swallowing, you should attempt to remove any food that is still in the mouth safely.

Seek advice from their physician if the person you are caring for is having trouble breathing or choking while eating or drinking; a speech and language therapy evaluation could be necessary.

Consult their physician if they're having problems swallowing pills or a local chemist who can help.

How to assist them when they put too much food in their mouths

If the person you care for is overeating, you can do a few things to help them.

A gentle touch on the arm accompanied by a gentle reminder to "take your time"; cutting all food into small pieces before serving it; encouraging the person to eat slowly and in small mouthfuls; using smaller cutlery, like a teaspoon or dessert fork; Cramming food into one's mouth puts one at risk of choking. Seeing someone with dementia choke on their meal can be frightening.

Changing behaviors at mealtimes

As dementia progresses, an individual may show behavioral abnormalities at mealtimes.

Understanding Changes in Mealtime Behaviour

Memory changes, as well as eating and drinking. Dementia patients frequently have difficulty staying seated at a table and paying attention throughout a meal.

How to assist with eating and drinking at mealtimes.

If alterations in behavior are impacting eating and drinking, then some interventions may be helpful.

Some of these interventions are:

- Encouraging them to take the initial bite to obtain a flavor.

- Make recommendations by saying something like "That's nice"

- Try a few mouthfuls of liquid first, then go to the spoon if they open their lips more readily to a cup than to a spoon.

- Encouraging them to eat as much as they can by themselves, regardless of how messy it is.

- Try a variety of flavors and textures; people who are suffering from dementia usually like sweet dishes. You can use sugar, ketchup, or maple syrup to sweeten your cuisine.

If they consume dangerous foods or insufficient amounts of nourishment, they may become susceptible to several ailments. People who have dementia may experience more confusion as they get worse.

SAFETY CONCERNING NON-FOOD ITEMS

A person with dementia may confuse household objects for food as the condition progresses.

They could try to eat liquid tabs, buttons, or tissues. They could hurt themselves as a result of this.

You can take certain precautions to avoid this.

Here are a few instances:

- Making sure all caregivers, including guests, are aware of this; and storing all hazardous materials, such as cleaning supplies, out of reach.

- Staying vigilant and taking out little objects that are readily ingested

- Offer food in place of the item as they could be hungry

- To ensure that kids can safely eat whenever and whatever they want, make sure food is available and easily accessible throughout the day.

How to Respond to Changes in Food Preferences

A person with dementia could start to prefer sweeter foods. As much as you can, give them a range of meals.

Among the items that might be beneficial are:

- Adding sugar to food before or after cooking; savory dishes can benefit from the sweet taste of honey, jam, syrup, and fresh fruit.

- Adding sugar to food before or after cooking; fresh fruit, honey, jam, and syrup can all be used to add sweetness to savory recipes.

- Playing around with savory dishes that are already sweet, such as sour and sweet sauces, pig and apple in cider sauce, barbecue sauces, gammon and pineapple, coated in honey, and sweeter curries. Adding strong-tasting condiments to food, such as ketchup or sweet chili sauce - these should be tried in tiny amounts to determine likes and dislikes. Enhancing tastes with herbs and spices

- If the person does not like strong-flavored dips, such as garlic mayo or barbecue sauce, use them instead.

CHAPTER FIVE

DEMENTIA PATIENTS CAN BENEFIT FROM FINGER FOODS AND EXERCISES

Nutritional and hydration issues are common complaints associated with dementia. One strategy that can increase total food intake and prolong the period of time that people with dementia can feed themselves is the use of finger foods.

What foods are finger foods exactly?

Foods that are small enough to be picked up with one hand and don't need cutlery are known as finger foods.

Eating with freedom and dignity is made possible by handheld foods, which also help to increase meal acceptance. When preparing finger foods, make sure the options are simple and enticing.

A Selection of Finger Meals for People with Dementia and Those Who Provide Care for Them.

To help you provide diversity and a balance of nutrients throughout the day, this list is divided into food groups.

While it's acceptable that nutrition won't be ideal for people with dementia, the best general guideline is to aim for 3-5 food types every meal.

Finger Foods Made of Starches and Grains

- Bagels in small or regular slices
- Biscuits with jam
- Soft cereal bars
- Crackers
- Croissants
- English muffins
- French toast sticks
- Fries
- Granola bars that are chewy rather than crumbly
- Little cinnamon rolls
- Mini donuts
- Mini muffins
- Halved new potatoes
- Pancakes either plain or with syrup to dip
- Pasta either plain or with sauce to dip

- Potato wedges

- Pretzel nibbles

- Ravioli either plain or with sauce to dip

- Sweet potato fries

- Tater tots and

- Toast, quartered or strips.

Finger Foods Using Vegetables and Fruits

- Mug-sized applesauce

- Peeled and chopped apples

- Whole or chunky bananas

- Blueberries

- Broccoli florets

- Broccoli - cheese tots

- Cauliflower florets

- Carrots, either raw or cooked

- Smoothie made with fruit

- Cut fruit with peel on (easy to hold)

- Halved grapes (caution: choking danger)

- Pineapple pieces

- Green beans

- Orange slices

- Pear slices with peels

- Watermelon sticks with the skin on them

- Deconstructed salad with dressing to dip

- Pureed fruit in a cup

- Raw veggies with or without a dip

- Strawberries cut in half

Finger Foods High in Protein

- Nuggets of chicken and boiled eggs, quartered

- Cubed chicken

- Sandwiched with chicken

- Chicken tenders, or split into big pieces and served on a bun

- Edamame (straight from the pod)

- Fish sticks

- Meatballs (little or half-sized)

- Deli meat (rolled up or in a sandwich)

- Mini quiche

- Rotisserie chicken

- Peanut butter (spread on crackers or sandwiches)

- Tiny or chopped sausage, tuna patties, and

- Salmon patties are some examples of mini burgers or sliders.

Finger Foods Contains Milk

Cheese cubes, cheese slices, cheese rolls, milkshakes, yogurt-based smoothies, string cheese, yogurt tubes, and drinkable yogurt and Kefir beverage.

Combinations of Finger Foods

- Pizza - bite-sized or cut into small squares

- Quesadilla - cut into triangles

- Sandwich - halves or quarters

- Smoothie

- Burrito

- Eggrolls

- Grilled cheese - quarters or; Kebabs - removed from skewer

- Peanut butter & banana wrap – sliced

- Mini cinnamon rolls

- Mini donuts

- Mini brownie squares or pieces

- Mini or regular cookies

- Ice cream bars

- Ice cream cones

- Ice cream sandwiches

- Milkshakes

- Popsicles

- Pound cake in cubes or strips, and

- Smoothies

ACTIVITIES AND EXERCISE FOR PEOPLE WITH DEMENTIA.

Engaging in suitable activities can assist an individual suffering from dementia in discovering purpose and enjoyment. Having fun doesn't require having a good memory. Many things provide us with delight and purpose every day. A person suffering from dementia still needs to live a high-quality life, but it is harder for them to do so when family members and caregivers are not there to support them.

There are several ways to organize and provide activities that are suitable for those who have dementia.

In an ideal world, activities would:

- Make up for lost abilities
- Boost self-esteem
- Preserve existing skills without demanding new ones; and
- Offer chances for enjoyment, fulfillment, and social interaction.
- Take the person's cultural background into account.

Organizing activities for people suffering from dementia

Having a thorough understanding of the dementia patient can help you organize activities that are suitable for them. This includes finding information about the individual's prior way of life, work history, interests in hobbies and other pastimes, past travel experiences, and significant life events. Avoid giving a person with dementia too much stimulation. Pick carefully what you go somewhere. Steer clear of noisy environments, crowds, and nonstop activity since they might overwhelm those who have dementia.

An activity care plan may be helpful if the individual is receiving care from numerous people. By doing this, you can make sure that the activities are suitable and consistent for the individual who has dementia.

Activities could contribute to restoring old roles.

Utilize forgotten abilities, including how to wash dishes, butter bread, or water, sweep, and rake the garden. These are other ways that the person with dementia might feel useful and contribute to the home. Urge them to assume some responsibility, however small.

Activities can provide both rest and enjoyment.

A dementia patient may enjoy a trip even though they are unable to remember where they have been. Even if the experience is soon forgotten, it is important to cherish the moment.

The most enjoyable hobbies are easy and leisurely. Give them adequate time and room to do as much as they can

SPLITING DOWN TASKS INTO MANAGEABLE SECTIONS.

Establish a safe working space

Patients suffering from dementia often have trouble with their vision and their balance. Keep surfaces clean and create as little noise and distractions as you can. Important factors to take into account include sitting choices, appropriate work heights, and good lighting (without glare). Make use of plastic containers to prevent breakage.

Don't let activities perpetuate inadequacies or stress you out. Ability levels might fluctuate from day to day. If activities were not successful or pleasurable the first time, they can be changed and tried again.

Utilize the number of hours that best suits the person's capacity for function.

To maximize performance when performing tasks, take into account the times of day when the person is most productive. For instance, it's occasionally ideal to walk in the morning or early afternoon. For those who feel restless later in the day or who have had an extremely long or pointless day, a late afternoon stroll could be more appropriate.

Promote an emotional connection

Many people with dementia are still able to move and feel rhythm. Dancing, connecting with infants, kids, or animals, or listening to music may all make you feel good.

People who are suffering from dementia often have excellent recollections of the past; looking through old pictures, books, and mementos may help the person remember the past.

It may be immensely satisfying to be able to go back and recall memorable moments. If their reading comprehension has declined, record them. Look for publications and picture books regarding the person's hobbies.

Incorporate pleasurable sensory sensations.

The following are some sensory experiences that a person with dementia might find enjoyable: getting a massage on their hands, neck, or feet; brushing their hair; smelling fresh flowers or pot pouring; using essential oils and fragrances; petting an animal or different-textured materials; going to a flower show or herb farm; or rummaging through a box filled with items that the person has shown interest in.

You can control tough behaviors with the aid of activities.

When it comes to managing harmful habits, activities are crucial. It's important to know what calms or distracts agitated or restless individuals. For caregivers on respite, this is quite helpful.

Most of all, never give up. Although mistakes and setbacks are inevitable, the individual suffering from dementia shouldn't feel inadequate.

EXERCISE AND DEMENTIA

Exercise has the same positive effects on persons with Alzheimer's disease as it does on healthy people in general, including increased cardiovascular fitness, strength, and endurance. A person should always get medical advice before starting any new exercise routine.

There are several health advantages to exercise, including:

- Better mood; better quality of sleep

- Decreased risk of constipation

- Preservation of motor skills

- Decreased risk of falls due to enhanced strength and balance

- Decreased rate of disease-associated cognitive decline

- Enhanced memory

- Improved behavior, including decreased rates of yelling, wandering, and aggressive behavior

- Enhanced social and communication skills.

Getting Started with A Physical Fitness Regimen.

Starting a fitness program for a patient with dementia might be recommended by the following:

- Speak with the patient's physician and set up a thorough physical examination. Certain medical conditions, such as high blood pressure or arthritis, may restrict the kinds of activities that a patient with dementia can safely perform.

- Based on the patient's current abilities and state of health, a physiotherapist can design an exercise regimen.

- Take it gradually at first. For instance, it's possible that initially, the person can only work for five minutes straight. Over a few months, increase the time by one minute at a time until the person can work out for 30 minutes without discomfort.

- Ask them to imitate you by doing the exercise yourself.

- To avoid becoming uninterested and losing drive, switch up your work periodically.

ACTIVITIES / EXERCISES FOR DEMENTIA SUFFERERS

If the individual used to like a certain type of activity, like golf, urge them to pick it up again with your support. Other suggestions are:

- Walking, which is a free and excellent all-around workout. Alzheimer's patients who walk also benefit from a reduction in their restless wanderlust. It might be advantageous to combine the stroll with a useful task, like taking the dog for a walk or running to the shop for milk.

- Cycling: Using a tandem bike allows you to ride in the front while your companion pedals from the back seat. Try renting a three-wheeled bicycle for the dementia sufferer to ride while you pedal behind them if they have problems staying balanced.

- Exercise apparatus

- Gym equipment such as treadmills, stationary bikes, and weight machines

- Aerobics - you may take classes together or rent low-impact aerobic workout videos.

Engaging in physical activity without feeling like it

Exercise is defined as any physical activity that causes an increase in heart rate. Some of the things to do that don't seem like organized exercise are:

- Dancing – Senior societies usually include dancing events into their social schedules. Even if the dementia sufferer is unable to dance, they can still learn and enjoy simple dances like square dancing.

- Gardening: raking leaves and cutting grass are excellent forms of physical activity. Ascertain that you are prepared to help if required.

- Housekeeping tasks, such as folding washing, and dusting. Most people with Alzheimer's disease may still perform some chores if they are closely watched.

Concerns about dementia patients' safety

Exercise can be beneficial for those with dementia, but exercises must be safe.

- As the patient's health worsens, discuss appropriate activities with the physiotherapist and doctor.

- Make sure the person wearing outside activities has on a medical alert pendant or bracelet and some sort of identification in case they get lost or stray off.

- If the individual is in a comfortable aerobic state, they should be using weight machines rather than droppable dumbbells or barbells. Continue talking to find out how inflated they are. Reduce the speed if they are unable to talk without gasping.

- When participating in outdoor activities, make sure the individual is sun savvy by wearing clothing, a hat, and sunscreen on all exposed skin regions.
- Check each drink on its own.
- Ensure that the person consumes adequate water before, during, and following exercise.
- Stop the activity and seek medical attention if the person reports feeling lightheaded, faint, or in pain.

CONCLUSION

A degenerative condition that limits a person's ability to live freely is dementia. There are several types of dementia, with Alzheimer's disease being the most prevalent. Before diagnosing dementia, a thorough assessment should be carried out as delirium and depression might be mistaken for the disease.

The aggressive actions that persons with dementia sometimes exhibit is not intentional; rather, they are the result of brain degeneration and are difficult for family members and professional caregivers to manage. Unfulfilled needs may give rise to difficult behaviors, which might function as a means of expression. By carefully observing what occurs just before and after the problematic behavior, the caregiver may be able to identify the underlying need and acquire strategies for calming it down.

Individuals with dementia need to be treated with compassion and a reminder that they are still capable of enjoying life. Physical and chemical limitations should be used as a last resort. Individualized therapy does not have to be limited by pharmacological and physical limits because many other options have been shown effective by science.

Dementia sufferers have disruptions in their daily routines. Family members and caregivers must intervene to assist with personal care and household management as dementia progresses. Activities, both solo and group, can improve people's self-esteem and quality of life.

Caregiver education ought to be provided to all those tending to a dementia patient. Especially in the early to moderate stages of the disease, family caregivers play a crucial and perhaps undervalued role in providing care for loved ones suffering from dementia. Stress is something that caregivers often experience, and it doesn't go away just by checking their loved one into a facility. Professional caregivers at a facility need to be taught to consider the individual with ADRD within the framework of their family.

Facilities that prioritize the needs of their residents can significantly and favorably impact harmful behaviors linked to dementia. It has been demonstrated that giving dementia patients a clean, safe, and homey environment where residents and staff work together improves their results.

When providing care for an individual with dementia, caregivers—both family and professional—face several moral conundrums. One of the most important strategies for enhancing the dementia experience is education and training in moral decision-making and conflict resolution.